Great Health

By Decision

Great Health
By Decision

Egil Nelius

How restoration
of my personal integrity
removed
long term issues

ISBN: 9781092846011

This is my story of how I restored my personal integrity and forgot what it meant to be sick, depressed, unmotivated, sexless.

Your integrity problems may be different from mine. But I hope that my story will nevertheless give you plenty of food for thought. So you can adapt those ideas to your own situation and needs, and start getting the best out of what the life has for you in store.

My most heartfelt gratitude to my wife Sandra, son Dag, friend Irita Logina

Disclaimer

The utmost care has been taken to accurately describe all the ideas, facts and attitudes.

However, the information in this book is not an advice and should not be treated as such.

For any actions that you might take inspired by the information presented here, you assume full responsibility of your own.

Real integrity is doing the right thing, knowing that nobody will know whether you did it or not.

Oprah Winfrey

With integrity, you have nothing to fear since you have nothing to hide.

With integrity, you will do the right thing, so you will have no guilt.

Zig Ziglar

If you have integrity, nothing else matters.

If you don't have integrity, nothing else matters.

Alan K.Simpson

Contents

Homework Before Visiting The Doctor

Here is the three of us - me (the doctor), you and the illness. Whose side you take, that party will win.

This quote of Avicenna, I saw in a doctor's office. Avicenna is a celebrated doctor of the ancient world who lied the early foundation of the medicine that we have nowadays.

It made me think. A funny question struck me. When we go to visit a doctor, do we always go there for - health? Do we always side with the doctor in the battle against the illness? Or are we most often the unaware allies of the illness, and go to the doctor only because it gives us the feel like taking an action?

If you fail to do your homework, if you shun your part of the responsibility, then you will get anything but health. You can get a false impression of an action, a temporary alleviation of the symptoms. But the most juicy and sexy outcome might be a grand show of the sequences of tests and investigations.

Tests and investigations, as a rule, will result in a therapy or surgery plan that targets the consequences while the cause remains unrevealed. For those who enjoy this kind of masochism, that must be a good news, because it promises for them a lot of repeated rounds of the "pleasure" of this kind.

But I personally see it as a nightmare, the worst of its kind. When I only think of it, I feel sick to the point that I can throw up.

When it comes to surgeries in particular, I am a terrible coward. I feel absolutely dead terrified at a thought that something might be cut and removed from my body, or, just opposite, a man made gadget planted into it.

What is even worse, I would have to live the rest of my life knowing it. I would become dependent on a medicine to compensate for the functionality of the removed organ. And, worst of all, I would still know that the root that caused this hazardous vivisection remains unremoved. And while the root cause is not found, chances are high that new ripping up and cutting would be needed again and again. The idea alone gives me the terrible ice cold creeps.

No, thank you. I'd rather go and do my homework.

And I did.

I took all the necessary measures to restore my personal integrity, and I took also a firm decision not to compromise it ever again.

For ten billion dollars, I would not give it up. I mean it.

I never knew that the life with integrity can be so enjoyable. I feel joy again. My health problems are all gone. I would never agree to go back to my old miserable existence, not even for ten billion dollars.

My personal integrity is of much greater value than what all the world's money can buy. My happiness, my good health, my inspiration, they all can exist only on the solid foundation of integrity. If it is lost, all is lost. That is why I won't ever sell it, whatever the price offer might be.

It is important to remember though, that I never aimed any health improvement or anything else healthwise. It just came without asking or calling when I chose to be a whole person. The curve having once run only down had turned determinedly to run upward.

And it was even not like checking the improvement on daily basis. Not at all. I was just living the life - working hard, drinking and savoring wine, noticing and savoring beautiful moments. I tried to always feel grateful until gratefulness became an integral part of my nature.

I allowed myself to feel pleasure and separated it determinedly from the sense of guilt, leaving the sense of guilt off board. I started to welcome pleasure in my life and stopped to regret it. I feel like what Kahlil Gibran's Prophet says: "...giving and receiving pleasure is both a need and a bliss."

My life changed. Eventually, it started to feel like really living, and has been like that ever since. Only occasionally a question occurred, like, where is my old life companion bronchitis! Does not seem like having visited for a number of years!

The Missing Piece In Wellness Advice

It would be great if any commercial piece of information regarding health and wellness contained a word of caution saying that, whatever we offer you to buy, will work only if you live with integrity.

Likewise, no matter what your success is, what you win or how much money you earn, it will give you true joy only if you do all things with integrity. Only people with integrity can feel true joy, the healing type of joy.

Joy is healing. Who did not know that? For whom that's a news? Nowadays, that's even proved scientifically. But where and how often do we see that stated, promoted explicitly? How often do we see people putting their trust in this simple yet universal and unavoidable principle? And how many of us ever come to an action? And how many are those who convert that trust and action into a lifestyle?

Do doctors advise patients to restore their integrity first, and only then come for help? Do diet consultants, oculists, psychotherapists and other health experts do? Do TV commercials that promote food or dietary supplements tell us clearly enough that they will give us a lasting improvement only if our integrity is undamaged?

Maybe they don't need to, because it should be considered a widely known, underlying, self-evident reality. But is it as a matter of fact?

Or do they, after all, get into the conflict of interests? The worst thing they fear is that you might get your health restored without the help of their product, their pill. Sure, they all want your health to improve. Somewhat, but not too much. Best of all, if you find how to maintain your (rather) good health by using their product. Then they are happy.

But what if you get your health restored just by changing your attitude, your way of thinking? And what if it gets restored completely? And what if it happens without their pill or diet plan? It means losing you as a paying customer, doesn't it? What business would want that? Which business can nowadays afford that at all?

Sure I want stability. Sure I want those companies to continue being profitable. But what I want still more is strong and happy people.

3

That is why I share with you …

… not a method, not a secret, not a wisdom, not a plan …

What I share with you is my faith in being only one person in one body. That is the attitude that gave me back my life, passion and - great health.

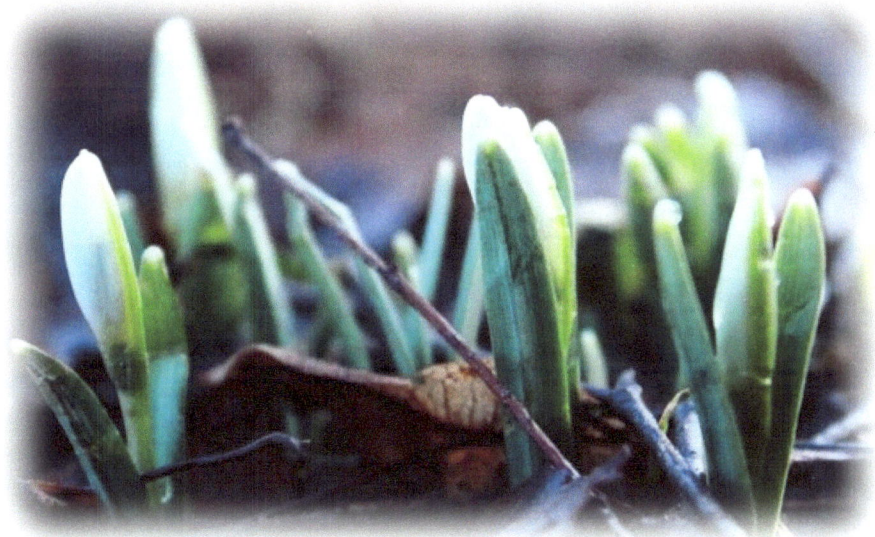

The One Thing That Separates Success from Failure

Whenever I see somebody wasting their efforts in a hopeless battle for health, chasing pills, therapies, diet plans, I try to encourage them to take the responsibility in their own hands. I tell them my own story of how my restored integrity alone helped me to improve my health and overall condition to a point of an incredible quality.

Whatever method or technique we may discuss regarding motivation, health improvement, mindful living, savoring of life, it will work only and exceptionally if our personal integrity is undamaged.

We seldom mention that explicitly. The authors who write on this subject are often unaware themselves. This is also a very delicate subject, and you always risk to become unpopular whenever you touch on it.

But the role of personal integrity can't be overestimated. It's role is always crucial. It is like having your ID document when you travel abroad. It is like having a ball in a soccer game. Because no traveling will happen without your ID document, and no soccer game will ever take place without a ball.

Too Accustomed To Even Notice The Problem

I would say even further and even more. If our integrity is damaged, we are not living the life. We are just - suffering it. We simply do not pay attention to the absolutely amazing reality. We do not celebrate the totally mind blowing fact that we are alive! Seldom or never it comes to our mind that the very fact that we hold the gift of life is in itself a mind blowing revelation. Isn't it as obvious as only can be? How come that it is taken seriously by too few? Yet it is.

The sad news is that too many people are so accustomed to living the life with damaged integrity that they don't even feel or know what they are actually missing. They want to be healthy, slim, strong, happy. They take therapies, slimming plans, they torture themselves with diets and workouts that they hate.

Then, after a day or two, or, OK, in the end of the week they stand before a mirror to check the result. When they realize that, instead of the hoped for huge improvement, there is nearly nothing to account for, then they will either give it all up right there or dive again in the ocean of information in a quest for a next plan or program, a more "efficient" one. And so they are caught in the vicious circle. Their rat race just goes on and on.

Is there a way to break this circle? Yes, absolutely.

Restored personal integrity will do the trick. On the one hand, the pills, therapies, plans that did not work before, may start being incredibly efficient all of a sudden. On the other hand, you may not even need those measures. Integrity, or call it being yourself, is a value of its own. Things can start getting sorted all by themselves.

Integrity As A Homework

Just complete your homework. Restore your integrity, and you will see all of a sudden that even those rejected plans and programs work well enough, even for you! More to that, you may soon notice that your condition is improving even when you are not using any program or pill at all.

When years ago I did just that, my overall health started to improve. It felt like healing all through my body. I never had it as a target. I never even gave that improvement any thought at all. It was much later that I noticed this unexpected change in my health. I just tried to recall my last time of being unwell, and it appeared in time somewhat before the point where I consciously changed my attitude.

It would be, after all, quite difficult not to associate it with all the immediate benefits that became available at that time. I feel stability like having the both feet of mine on a solid ground. I feel joy and amazement - for just being alive! And I feel inside myself how that joy is responsible for the healing "juices" that I now feel flowing all through my body.

Consequences of Neglecting

I see too many people these days who neglect their integrity. They miss out on feeling the joy of life, the joy of themselves being alive. They cause damage to their overall health by allowing poisonous "juices" to flow. The life itself that we have received as a generous gift, becomes an endless suffering.

What would be, after all, a single valid reason for anybody not to seize that joy, not to restore their integrity, not to treat their integrity with the due respect? Can there be any reason for anyone at all to be missing out on their life truly lived? Is it not easy as can be, obvious and natural for everyone? At times, a doubt comes over me as I write all this - for whom, actually, I write? Can there be a thing simpler and more obvious? Is there a single person in the whole world who would not understand?

But, hey, where are all those happy, generous, humble, grateful people who draw their inspiration directly from the amazing reality in which all of us exist? Why do we see instead so many crippled lives, so many people full of dissatisfaction and hate, so many of those who do not know what love is, what joy is, what sincerity is? Why do we see so many of them every day?

Something must be terribly wrong. But what? Can the real cause be identified? What is the wrong, blocking thing that makes us feel miserable in the middle of a fantastic, wonderful world? Why are we so unable to see the reality? How can it be that we are not amazed when we see the tremendous reality with ourselves being part of it? How can it be that we don't actually see what we see? How come that we miss out on enjoying the infinite number of miracles that are all placed right before our eyes?

A Myth That Blocks Action

There is a cause for all action being blocked. And that is a devilishly cunning one, that is even more difficult to spot simply because it usually is – too visible, too close to be even noticed. It may even pretend being a natural part of ourselves. It can be inside us, and may have been there for some time, long enough for us to get so accustomed that we don't feel any wrong at all. Yet they are all just "foreign bodies" in our soul, and only pretend to be part of it.

Things like guilt, resentment, unforgiving, hate, judgmental attitude, discontentment are "foreign bodies". None of them will ever be natural, integral part of ourselves. They often pretend to be, but that is a myth.

At times it may even seem that, if we remove them, we stop being our real selves. We may feel them as a natural part of ourselves and can't imagine our life with those removed. It may even be easier for us to imagine our future life without a kidney or a lung than to imagine it without any one of those long nourished enslaving attitudes that break our integrity and block us from seeing the reality. But that is just the other side of the same myth.

When we stay too long in this state, we lose the ability to love, and we start thinking that love does not exist. We are unable to feel true joy, and we start believing that there is only sorrow everywhere. We see injustice and we become part of that injustice ourselves thinking that being honest would do us wrong. That too is just a myth.

It is very important to take it in once and for eternal time: the above things and similar **are never part of the personality of any human being**.

Another myth, equally dangerous, is the one that now you need to identify the culprits each separately and spend an amount of time and efforts to weed them out. Some religions will present this myth as battling against sin in a battle that never ends.

Never fall for that. Don't ever get deceived by such a lie!

All you need to do is very simple. You need to fall in love, deeply and passionately, with your own self and with the life as such. You need to allow that warm shower of love to flow in and through yourself. You need to immerse yourself completely in it. And that is very easy, indeed. That is just a decision, the following of which is pleasant and rewarding.

Never focus on the culprits, demons, sins or whatever you may want to call them. Focus instead on love. And, first of all, on deep, unconditional love to your own self.

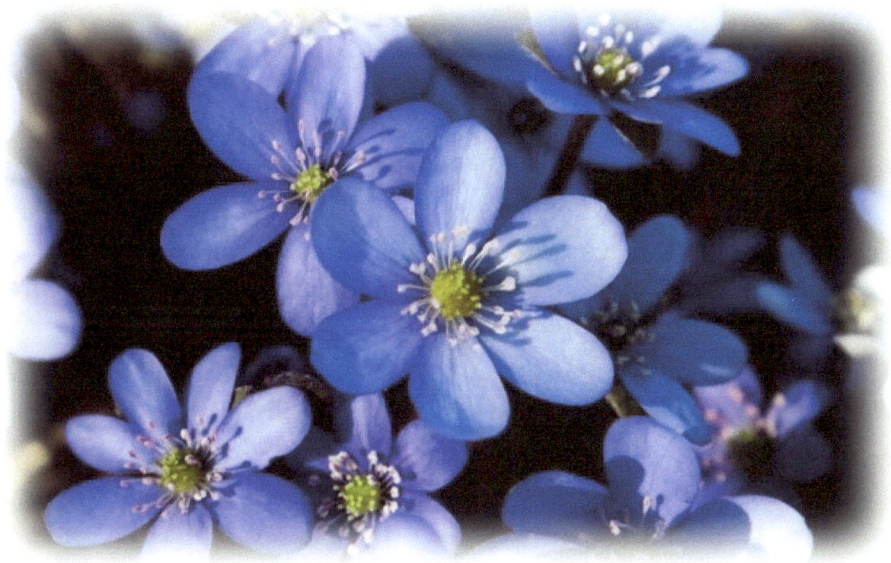

Aggressive Disintegrity

It may be hard even to believe, but there are people who would eagerly defend and justify their continued living with broken integrity. They would say that that is a part of their personality, of being their real selves!

I have met such people face to face, so I know what I am speaking of. They are, as a rule, under some damaging influence of a tradition, religion, pseudo science, biased education, whatever. And their fear to decide and cut it once and forever is paralyzing. These people can't even be helped before they take the decision for themselves.

Difference Between Personal Qualities And Things That Break Integrity

I mean to say that broken integrity is never an integral part of a person's real self. It is rather a factor that keeps them from being their real selves and living up to their real potential.

But how to distinguish, after all, what is and what is not a part of human personality and uniqueness? This might be a legal question, after all?

The answer should be rather obvious. Yours are your likes and dislikes, your talents and weaknesses, your victories and failures, your interests, your skills, etc.

But the state of being unhappy, depressed, sickly is never part of your personality. Being at war with yourself is not a part of yourself. Sense of inferiority of any kind is not and can never be an integral part of your own self. Any attitude that works against you as a full value person is not a part of yourself, no matter how deep it sits in your soul, and no matter how deeply accustomed you are to the slavery of that kind.

Guilt Without Guilt

Modern people often nourish sense of guilt in themselves which has nothing to do with any real guilt. At times, I get speechless when I hear for what people can deem themselves guilty!

"When I catch myself by the refrigerator in the middle of the night taking our fat food and eating it, I shame myself, yet keep eating," says a woman in a magazine article.

"I feel guilty for not being able to give birth to a healthy child," said a Mother of a sick baby.

Are these not loud enough examples of how cunning the sense of guilt can get at times? And these are not just some singular instances. This attitude of self shaming is widely promoted in media. Social networks are full of it, too.

Please notice, here are, in fact, two persons in one body. The "good you" catches the "bad you" doing something indecent, something shameful. And that "good you" then accuses the "bad you".

People feel guilty for eating, for resting, for having called you when you are busy, for not being married, for being married, for not having children, for not being able to have them, for having too many children, for being overweight, for being underweight, for even being alive.

But how often do we consider what the very sense of guilt does to our personality, to our health.

Right here and now, you should stop feeling guilty for natural things and things that are beyond our control.

Love yourself instead, and love the life with the full wholeness of your heart. Always remember to feed yourself on joy and pleasure. Those have incredible healing power.

Guilty For Being Sexual

A specific and very disastrous kind of sense of guilt is the one for being sexual, for feeling and living sexually. Unfortunately, this type of inspired guilt is heavily promoted and stimulated by traditions, religions, even legislation.

Some countries have very harsh laws on human sexuality. The lawmakers just issue laws on things that are given to people by nature, not by a will of man. There are too many rules that do not remove from people their sexual nature, but only make them feel guilty for it. There are too many humiliating words by which sexuality is referred to.

It is easy to manipulate with sexually dissatisfied people. For example, religious extremists know that only embarrassed people can be turned into blind followers, even suicide bombers. That is why they do everything to keep their people in that mental state. They know that they can not manipulate with people of integrity, and that such people can potentially be a threat for their system, their positions, their income.

That way, personal integrity is connected with courage. Aggressive systems and those who control them will often try to target your sexuality in order to plant the sense of guilt in you, and, ultimately, break your integrity. People who believe that they are guilty, are easily controllable. They can be trained literally into anything, even mass murderers. There are regions on our planet where being and staying your true self requires enormous courage and determination, even under the threat of life.

So, where to get the courage needed? How to be brave enough to always be your real self? How not to give in to fear? How to be able to stand under the pressure that at times may come even from the closest people?

How to stay whole when the world around you seeks to break you?

Some time tested sources of courage you will find lower in this book.

Reasons For Attachment To A Brainwashed State

No wonder that the bosses of the aggressive systems will do everything to protect their system. They will try to present all the sound people as fools, sinners, enemies. Some systems will even kill them. And it is rather easy to understand why it happens. The bosses themselves as well as their systems do have something to lose. So they will always direct their hate and all their power against those who question the usefulness of those systems.

But there is also the other side. The indoctrinated people themselves will actively defend their state of being indoctrinated. They are prepared to fight even though they feel miserable. The more miserable, in fact, they feel, the angrier they get with those who refuse to be indoctrinated.

They may have access to only a tiny part of all the benefits if any at all. What the leverage could be then that has the power of keeping them in that brainwashed state?

When I researched a little, I found these three reasons. First of all, that is insufficient faith, insufficient trust in what they feel deep inside. Second, it will be fear from the system, and the third will be their fear that the change of their attitude would require also a change of their lifestyle, of their ways and habits.

Lack Of Faith

It may not be easy to trust your own senses if you have been mistrusting them the whole life up to this point. But down with all doubts! Please start doing. Please reunite with yourself even if you have never been united! Nothing in the whole world can replace that wonderful condition of being one with your own self.

On the other hand, if you are not, you are exposed to all the evils. Too many people live like two hostile persons within the same body. Depression, illnesses, obesity, broken relations, addictions – they all basically stem from the same root. Failure to unconditionally accept yourself, failure to forgive, failure to let go a trauma and similar things,

14

those are all, well, I can't say, risks. Those are, every single one of them and collectively, direct causes for awful suffering, for a life not lived.

Your only option, only way to go is a complete and unconditional self acceptance. No more cyanide in the honeypot! No more excuses! Your personal integrity is the basis for all your wellness. This is where you start.

System Fear

System fear should not keep you from action. When I say, system, it can mean not only a political or religious system. It can be even your own family, your circle of friends.

They can all get upset seeing your independence and feeling the weight of your will. Especially, if you've been all the way just a puppet. How dare you now to be a person? Yes, you dare!

A loving family, good friends will understand and accept you as you are. In the final score, they will start truly enjoying the relationship with you. It feels different to receive friendship and love from somebody who is a person, and not a puppet!

All those who can't accept you being with integrity are not your friends. Don't change yourself because they require a change in you. Most likely, they will have to go from your life. Just allow them to go!

But don't lock yourself. To a degree possible, stay open for them, just in case. At a certain point, they may want to come back when they start honoring their own integrity. Then they will start respecting yours, as well. That would be a good news! Between self sufficient, undivided people, great relationships can potentially be established.

But vampires, they need to leave. At least until they turn away from their vampirish ways, become personalities themselves and learn to appreciate us being personalities.

Fear Of Change

Speaking about the habits, yes, it is true that some of them are incompatible with personal integrity. But it is not that you need to change your habits because you want to restore your integrity. For me it worked the other way round. First came the decision. I just decided to stop being

15

an enemy of myself and start being a friend. So some of my bad habits died naturally.

My habit of having low opinion about myself just discontinued naturally. I started to see how wonderfully works my mind and my body. I started learning new things. I started feeling valuable just as I am.

I learned to say Yes when I felt like Yes. I learned to say No when I felt like No. I now say "I don't know" when I don't know. I just stopped to manipulate my answers by guessing the expectancies. I am kind, I am friendly and polite. Only I don't say Yes anymore when I think differently. I don't adjust my opinion to what others might want to hear. Paradoxically, it is far from any hostility what I receive in exchange. What I receive is only respect and understanding.

We teach others how to treat us by showing them how we treat ourselves.

I had to change a number of habits, and I did. I feel that you too will have to deal with a number when you take the decision. But the good news is that the change is easy. That is a change towards what is natural, and that is why your own body will be your ally in that highly rewarding effort. No willpower involved, just a conscious permission for yourself to feel what you feel as a matter of fact. Just learn to trust what you actually feel and follow that feeling.

Just don't be deceived. You need to clearly distinguish between the habit and the natural desire of your body. For example, no matter how long you have been a smoker, your body does not want you to smoke. Love your body, and treat it with love.

Likewise, lack of movement will never be a thing that your body desires. Love yourself, respect yourself and take every chance to move. It is easy. Moving is easy. Keeping yourself attached to the sofa, that is the real torture. Your body would never vote for that.

It is snow in the forest now. Me and my friend, we went on a 7 miles or so walk. Every step required an effort. The snow was deep. Here and there under the snow, there were spots with slippery ice. In some other places, lumps of frozen soil and furrows left by some vehicle were under the snow. Frost was biting our cheeks.

But the funniest thing was that we did not feel any of that at all. We felt life flowing through us. We chatted, laughed, watched the beautiful views in the snowy forest. We felt happy.

Then in our conversation, we touched the subject of our own responsibility for seeing and feeling joy. We figured what the opposite might be. We tried to count the unfortunate things that might have stopped us from having our beautiful forest moments. And, yes, we found a number of them.

Every single one of them might have "served" us being a sufficient reason for not having the walk. It was too cold. It was too lumpy. It was too slippery. The snow was too deep.

Why did we not see and pay attention to any of these inconveniences from the beginning? Yes, because for some time already, we have been practicing seeing the good, the beautiful, the encouraging side of all things. Now we have already reached the point where it works for us effortlessly.

We did not notice, we did not pay any attention to the unfortunate things. Even the whole bunch of them went for us unnoticed.

We chose once to first see the advantages. Now we feel that this attitude has "grown" into us. We don't have to think and remember it anymore. It is like you learn driving just once, and then you know how to do it for the rest of your life.

We feel that the habit of seeing the advantages now sits deep in the marrow of our bone. But in the beginning, that was not as natural as it feels now. It required an effort not to focus on the barriers. But as we persisted practicing this attitude, it gradually changed even our subconscious.

Now our default attitude is - wow, what a beautiful walk! And those "unfortunate", difficult, challenging things, in a paradoxical manner, they just form a background on which our joy can shine even brighter.

So was that a change in me – shifting the focus from potentially blocking things to the joy of doing? Yes, it was. Was that a change towards my personal integrity, my personal wellness? Yes, absolutely. Was that a difficult change? Not at all. It required some courage, yes, it did. It required also breaking of some bad habits. But all in all, that was an easy change. It felt good, natural. The process of changing from suffering attitude to proactive attitude was highly enjoyable, too.

The most difficult part of all will most certainly be the very recognition to yourself that you have some bad habits, unproductive thinking patterns, blocking attitudes. Those need to be identified and removed.

Well, it is not that you need to identify every single one of those "giants". I just started actively finding and connecting to what gives me joy. When some joy started flowing in me, all those "giants" just left without any trouble at all.

But it can happen only if you recognize that there are those "giants" in you. And if you have them, it is dangerous to pretend that you don't. You may not attach yourself to them or harbor them. If you do, then you just won't be able to restore your integrity.

In any case, you have to be wise and absolutely honest with your own self.

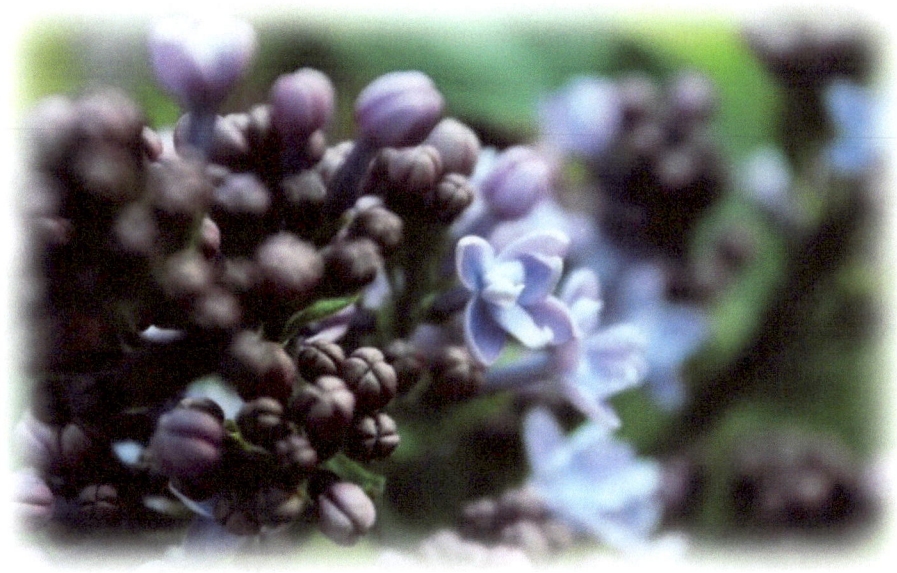

Joy And Bodily *Juices*

My First Encounter With The Joy

I remember the very first time when I felt that all-embracing joy flowing all through myself. Only some time later I realized that this experience was closely linked to my decision to live with integrity.

That was a sunset on a beach. Just one of the hundreds of sunsets that I had seen. But this one was very special, because it was the first one ever that I really SAW!

The fact of being alive, that red Sun, the astounding tapestry of the sunset sky and the ocean, all this felt so amazingly REAL!

I felt my heart beating. I felt the joy flowing. It tickled in my belly, it pulsated in my temple. I felt a strong urge to run and jump like mad. I wanted to shout and sing. The unexpected, sudden joy carried me like on wings.

If somebody saw me that moment, they may have thought that I was hopelessly drunk! But I was absolutely sober. More sober than ever before.

Since then, I have felt and experienced that joy many times. I have even started to notice that it does not leave me any more. It feels like it is constantly present and has found in me a place to dwell.

Why So Many Fail To Recognize The Joy

Will I surprise you by telling that, having experienced that joy, I wanted to share it with others. I spoke eloquently and enthusiastically. But in the eyes of my interlocutors, I did not see the light that I would have expected. Their eyes, to my great surprise, did not light up any at all. They did not, even if the shared news was exciting, uplifting, highly encouraging!

Did they not want to experience that all-embracing, intoxicating, inspiring, healing joy that I was speaking about? Were they not surprised to hear the message that such a joy at all exists? Were they totally unable to see how easy it was to immerse yourself into that reality based joy, fill yourself with it and enjoy all the benefits that it gives to you?

Did they think I was fantasizing or trying to preach a new religion? Did they think I was? Did they think anything at all?

Only one thing was very clear - they did not understand what I was talking about.

In any case, why did they not stand up and try it before they deemed me hopeless? It is so readily available for anyone, it is so real, so tangible. Just open your eyes, see the reality, the amazing reality and allow the joy to flow in your veins. That's all there is to it. You will see by yourself how real that is!

But then I gradually started to pick up the real reason for their being so negative. They had not done their homework yet. No person whose integrity is compromised in one way or the other, will ever be able to see the reality inspired joy, let alone enjoy it or benefit from it.

There should be no worries though. Restoring of the integrity is easy. It is even ridiculously easy. The life is much easier, in fact, when you live with integrity. In the most difficult moments, your integrity may become the true source of strength and endurance. In the heaviest moments, when everyone else would be down, you can still retain the cheerful frame of mind due to your being a whole and undivided person.

With integrity, even in the moments when I feel weak and tired, somewhere in the deepest deep I still feel the firm ground to stand on. In this paradoxical manner, even in the moments when I am terribly down, I know that soon I will be well again. And the very moment of being down is not that terrible as it might feel if I were miserable and wrecked on the inside.

But I am not. I am no longer. I have chosen my attitude and done that with determination. I have tasted once how easy and enjoyable it is to simply live by - reality. I like it, I love it, and I won't ever come back to my old foolish attitudes even if you pay me, even if you give me all the money of the whole world.

If you care, if you are a friend of your own self, then you should put in some effort to understand very clearly what I am trying to say here. If not, then, yeah, why are you reading at all?

Let me make a few bullet points.

» There is an all-embracing, healing, breathtaking joy in a mindful connection to the independent reality and feeling yourself part of it.

» Only the people who choose to live with integrity can feel that joy.

» That joy has the power to reverse your declining health, make inefficient therapies efficient, may even help you to live without any therapies at all.

» To get hold on that joy, you need to do your homework, which is restoring your integrity (please, read the next chapters) and connecting mindfully to the reality.

Controlling Of The *Juices*

You may have heard of a substance called Adrenaline that certain glands emit into our body when we face a challenge or are about to do something that requires a little courage.

Under certain conditions, the level of Testosterone will increase, which is a fluid, too.

There are fluids and things being emitted and used, that circulate in our body all of the time.

Thoughts And *Juices*

Depending on what we think, what ideas we allow in to our head, determines what kind of substances keep flowing in our body.

When we notice what is beautiful in the nature, when we feel grateful, when we feel in love, there will be one type of those substances flowing. But when, on the contrary, we are bitter, angry, revengeful, then the substances are different.

All this will make sense with realization of just this one simple idea – we all are the true masters of our thoughts. Ours is the responsibility, full and undivided, for the thoughts that are allowed in to our brain and soul. Our thoughts, the ideas in our head, they are made to obey us, and they do.

It is not a valid complaint if you try to say that you can't discipline your own thoughts. Yes, you can. It is you who decides what you think and what you don't. Thinking yourself out of an undesired condition into something that you can truly enjoy is nobody's business but yours.

Bitter, depressed thoughts trigger emission of poignant substances into your body. Whereas, bright, joyous thoughts generate sweet, pleasant juices. You decide what you want for yourself.

A widespread delusion is believing that the thoughts that we spin in our heads are dependent on our situation, on the outside conditions. In fact they are not. It is our will, not our situation, that has the power to influence our thoughts. It is us who decide what we think and, consequently, what *juices* we feed our body on. And that, in its turn, will determine our health and overall condition.

No one can stay healthy thinking bitter thoughts in a longer period of time. On the contrary, those who think happy thoughts are usually also happy themselves. But happy people are seldom sick. The decision is yours and yours alone.

Connection To The Independent Reality

Please don't ever use any kind of "positive thinking". Sometimes people get confused and think that that is exactly what I call for. But in fact I never do. Just opposite, I often try to warn people about the hidden dangers of thinking "positively".

The thing that I would suggest and encourage for everyone is staying connected. Connect to the very fact that you are alive. Is it not efficient enough, breathtaking enough? Look upon everything from that perspective. The life can be interrupted at any point, it is very fragile. But this very moment, you still hold it, and chances are that you will be holding it for many more years. But you don't have any promise.

The idea alone of being alive is powerful enough to make your heart rate increase. It can fill your body with excitement and joy. Keeping ourselves aware of the amazing fact that we hold the gift of life, should, strictly speaking, always be enough to keep us happy and cheerful.

But the problem is that we forget that too often. We forget everything – our identity, our roots. We fail to notice what we see. We seldom pay attention to the amazing world around us.

Everyday problems like giants besiege us. We feel scared, angry, depressed. We forget to focus on who we are and what we are as a matter of fact.

Bad, bitter streams flow through our bodies and souls. If we live like that for a longer period of time, how far is then depression and all those severe health problems?

Why don't we just lock out all those destructive streams from our being by simply stopping the unsubstantiated way of thinking? We are the masters of our thoughts. Let's take the responsibility in our own hands and fill ourselves with reality based ideas. So the junk will have to stay outside.

Being In Movement As Part Of Integrity

I heard a doctor present a recent discovery of the science. The bones of our body, the skeleton is capable of producing and emitting of a matchless medicine that works efficiently against a large number of serious illnesses, like diabetes, osteoporosis, and I think he mentioned even cancer.

To activate the production and emission of that "medicine", we need to ram, stretch and twist the bones. In other words, we need to move vigorously, intensively, without overprotecting joints or feet. The idea of the harm of overprotecting is supported explicitly in Cristopher McDougall's book "Born To Run".

Do I believe? Yes, I do. Because that message was nothing new to me. My personal experience in decades supports it. Movement is, after all, part and parcel of my integrity. I knew long since what also my dog knows and every little child feels and acts accordingly. To keep our body happy, we need to move, and move a lot!

More to that, we need to learn to enjoy the process. Not before, not after, but right in the middle of the movement, in the middle of the workout, we need to be able to enjoy it. And a good workout is highly enjoyable by its nature.

It is like a paradox again. Working your body hard is, in fact, easy and enjoyable. Not working your body, forcing yourself into sedentary lifestyle, that is what in fact is really difficult. That is a real self torture!

"I am too lazy!"

"I don't have willpower!"

Those are the stories that we hear day in day out. But is that so difficult to see that the real and true manifestation of true laziness is running, jumping, swimming, cycling, skiing, skating, weight lifting and all the other ways of moving, moving and moving? Our bodies need it, and it requires, in fact, a horrible effort to train our body to stay on the sofa when it thirsts for movement!

Even more difficult are the therapies and surgeries that are attracted, as a rule, by unused energy in our body. Our natural energy, if we keep it without its natural turnaround, becomes its opposite. It starts causing tiredness. Yeah, believe me or not, for a large part of our tiredness, the responsibility does not lie with exhaustion. Our tiredness can be often caused by the unused energy surplus. And, if we keep our sedentary manner for years, then it is very likely to start attracting all the worst kinds of illnesses, too.

That is the paradox. What is difficult is, as a matter of fact, easy. What seems easy, is, in reality, terribly difficult. I want the good *juices* to be running inside me, so I choose to move. And I move a lot. But, again, I don't move for the sake of those *juices*. I don't move for health. I move only, only, only because I truly and deeply enjoy being in movement.

And you, my reader, you may not believe me, but you too are one of them who truly enjoys being in movement. How do I know that? Well, because all humans are by their nature.

Hating movement is not natural. Sedentary lifestyle is not compatible with any person's integrity because it is not natural. All the people have the urge for movement nested deep in their being. All the people want moving, and they thirst for moving. All the people want to feel their muscles to endure a workload, all of them want to enjoy the restoring rest that only comes if the day has been lived and worked well.

Starving our body on movement is not a way of showing kindness. It is a terrible abuse, let all of us just take in this simple truth!

But there are those among us who have starved themselves on moving too long. They can't feel that drive anymore. But fear from movement is not natural. It is forced onto us by the multitude of modern gadgets that all are designed to make our life easier. But as a matter of fact, they only distort the idea about the joy of moving and the joy of taking physical challenges.

What can be done then? Well, you can do yourself a favor. Start off with just thinking of running, jumping, swimming, lifting and other sporty things like of being pleasant, enjoyable, rewarding. Move gradually forward. Shape that pleasantly expectant attitude. Meanwhile, start doing something. Move on little by little. Start gradually taking bigger challenges. Never set any goals. Let the only goal be – pleasure!

Do it, savor it, grow into it, feel the taste. A day will come soon when you realize that, hey, you just can't wait to run that flight of stairs again, the same one that you used to avoid by taking the elevator.

Sometimes, I can be too busy to go for a run or to start a workout. But I take the advantage of, for example, choosing to run where I would otherwise walk. Whenever I have a chance, I avoid elevators and run the stairs. Even when I sit and write, I try to remember to strain and release my abs, muscles in my shoulders, arms, legs. I thirst for moving until I reach a certain amount for the day. I use every chance to give my body the movements that it longs for.

It works really well for me. But I can only speak about myself. You need to test it and try it for yourself. Moving, and moving intensively, is natural. It does not cost you money unless you use a paid gym. It does not pose any threat greater than any other everyday activity. Yes, the life as such is not safe, is it?

Only be careful if you are just starting after a long period of being sedentary. Maybe consult your doctor then.

But normally, if you need a doctor's permission for moving, then you need one for living, as well. That is just getting too funny nowadays.

How To Describe Integrity

Integrity is often defined as honesty, a state of being a whole person. Good. It must be so at large. But I feel some building bricks that make that honesty and wholeness should be mentioned here, too. I will try to list a number of approaches or attitudes that are part of my own personal integrity.

I have studied a lot of materials on this subject and spoken to a lot of people, and I feel that, for most people, these attitudes work more or less in the same manner.

The list will come in two blocks. First, there will be the "decent", well-behaved, good looking attitudes. The other block will list some not so obvious, somewhat fierce, somewhat wild, somewhat counter-intuitive, often misinterpreted and often frowned at attitudes which are, nevertheless, equally important.

The Rather Well Behaved Attitudes

My personal integrity is full and unconditional acceptance of my own self.

My personal integrity is being my true self regardless of what others may think or say.

My personal integrity is holding full responsibility for my life, and not blaming anyone else.

My personal integrity is knowing that the life as such is not just, and being OK with that.

My personal integrity is the ability, or rather a decision to feel deep joy for other people's success and readiness to always assist them to their success, should it become dependent in a way on my support.

My personal integrity is complete forgiveness of all the wrongs ever done to me in the past, and even forgiving in advance all the wrongs that may come in the future.

My personal integrity is conscious "connecting" to the real world and finding joy in "ordinary" things.

My personal integrity is full freedom from sense of guilt, real or imaginary.

Empathy is an inseparable part of my personal integrity. Before I speak or act, I try to always remember to put myself in the shoes of those affected. I always try to a degree possible to act in a manner that would lift them up rather than beat them.

You can't bribe me, you can't buy my opinion. Not even for very big money. And not because I would be such a nice guy, excessively law obedient. Not at all. But you can't corrupt me because I simply respect my own self and value my integrity above all the things that money can buy.

At a certain point, I made an effort to foster in me the awareness of the elusive nature of human life. None of us will live forever. And where we go then, we cannot take a single penny with us.

And what if you are sent to that final journey tonight or tomorrow? Do you have any promise that you will be given a one more day tomorrow? What is the value of all your mansions and yachts when you measure it against this reality?

The Untamed Attitudes

I actively cultivate in me the awareness of my own mortality. I often think deliberately about death. That is a paradox again, but this awareness sets me free. It teaches me to appreciate the current moment since I can't know how many more of them I will be given. It removes all greed, jealousy, worries and similar things from my mind and life.

It reminds me of the need to live the life here and now, and fill it to a degree possible with love and joy. It gives me courage to be a man of action, because I always ask myself a question whether I would still stand irresolute if I knew that this day would be my last. And since it may also very well be, I better stand up and act.

It helps me to feel deep gratefulness for the current moment. It gives me humble mindset, so I am able to notice the beauty of this world.

It cuts all the strings that may have tied me to properties, luxuries, wealth, connections. Ironically, it enables me to truly enjoy all those things – much better than before. I am no longer their slave. I am their master now because I know their real value. I see that it is absolutely useless to worry about your next moment if it is only this current moment that truly belongs to you.

I don't use positive thinking of any kind. I do often use **negative visualization** and find it helpful. I imagine that what I value can be taken away from me in any moment. That boosts my ability to be grateful and to value the precious moments with my loved ones. I can see also that the right attitude is to be grateful for the moments that are given to me rather than feeling destroyed when my loved ones are no longer here.

When I visualize negative scenarios to a degree how bad they can get altogether, I see that none of them is quite as bad as they would seem at a first glance. When I prepare for unpleasant embarrassing situations, I find ways how I can feel good enough even when I have to go through them.

I don't take ultimatums. Whenever confronted with two ultimate options, I always choose the bad one, the threatening one. Not even once in my lifetime I have regretted that.

When I don't allow threats to influence me, I support my integrity. Apart of that, it is extremely rare that those threats come true as a matter of fact.

I don't give way to "scientific intimidation". Intimidating "scientifically proved" information is, unfortunately, our everyday. This product or that is bad for your health. Without this pill or that, you will die.

I have identified this "channel" and switched it off completely in my heart and mind.

Now, the scientists of the whole world may come to my doorstep carrying slogans saying that, let's say, milk is bad for my health. Boldly and shamelessly, I will continue using it and focus even more on the joy that it gives me.

And, yes, there are also "pills" without which I would die.

Some of my "pills" would be:

» gratefulness,

» being in love,

» true, deep, reality and sound reason based happiness, which is a happiness by choice,

» active, dynamic lifestyle,

» honesty in everything,

» generosity and similar enjoyable and uplifting things.

I need no other pill. Honestly.

Sometimes I break the rules, but never for the sake of just breaking them. This happens if e.g. a matter of greater importance is at stake. E.g. once I have a question to which I need an answer, the sign "Staff only" won't keep me from getting that answer.

In situations when the Law would require me to act against my integrity, I would always choose to stay with integrity even though that might be considered illegal from the point of view of the pervert law. Well, let me give you a harsh example.

In the countries that were under Nazi rule, it was a requirement to denounce on people of certain ethnicity. Many people did inform even on their friends and neighbors. Others were saving and hiding them, even at the risk of their own lives. Will it be difficult to answer which ones compromised and lost their integrity, and which were those who fortified it by acting bravely?

In the final score, it is always better even to die, but with integrity, than to continue the miserable existence having lost it. Because you may call your life Life (with the big capital letter) only if you live it with integrity. Whenever you give up your integrity, that is not life anymore. What it is then? I don't know. Hell, perhaps?

My personal integrity is also **complete freedom from jealousy**. I see all too often that loving "unconditionally" turns into extremely nasty business whenever the one you love has some nice moment with someone else. I had to cut that. When I love somebody, I try to do that truly unconditionally. Their joy is my joy, and their pleasure is my pleasure, even if that is not me giving them that joy in that particular moment.

Well, I read the other day that there was even a specific word in the English language to denote an attitude that is an opposite to jealousy. I don't remember and I don't care what that word was. It translated like the ability to feel joy when your loved ones feel joy.

That there is such a word, it is, no doubt, a huge step in the right direction. But I personally don't need it, because I see that the opposite of "jealousy" already exists. And that is "Love". It is not true that love has some small amount of jealousy in it. No. Love and jealousy are mutually excluding opposites. If you still want to add some portion of jealousy to your love, then you will get a similar end product as when you would add a tiny drop of cyanide to a keg of honey. The honey will become poison, won't it? In the same manner, love will stop being love. It will turn, in fact, into just ownership of the other person.

All too often I see that people treat each other as a property. They simply don't know what they are missing. They have long since lost all "spice" of their being together. Too many married people don't sleep in the same bed, or even in the same room. Some of them don't even talk to each other, and may have been like that for many years.

Why do they treat each other like that? Isn't the life too short and too wonderful for an attitude like that?

Birds in cages do not sing. There are only two options. If you want to hear them sing, then set them free. You can also choose to keep owning them. But then you should know that you won't ever hear them sing.

Zero jealousy and setting the other person free is the way how you start enjoying the true pleasure of being together. People often mistake me and my wife for being on our first date, because it is always quite obvious that we truly enjoy each other's company. They are surprised when they learn that we have been together for more than 30 years!

What is our secret, they would ask. Well, instead of spying on each other or finding guilt in each other, we choose to value and enjoy our moments of being together. There is really nothing more to that.

My attitude towards "serial monogamy" is like towards an ultimate cruelty. Breaking an existing relationship in order to start a new one is evil, cowardly, treacherous and plain stupid. I would never choose to be guilty of such.

This practice, however widely considered acceptable, will ruin your integrity the very moment when you just conceive the first tiny sprout of an idea. The first time when you even admit such a possibility, you are ruined. And it does not matter the least whether you use some pills or refrain from certain kinds of food. None will help you. None.

But the things once done cannot be undone. What if you have divorced your heart and soul and married somebody "better"? How to cope with the wrong decision once taken? Is there a way of clearing that guilt?

Well, then you need to forgive yourself truly and completely, and once and for all times. Just forgive yourself and commit yourself to repairing whatever can still be repaired!

I am not speaking here about the situations when being in legal bound is a torture, when there is long since no actual relationship. I speak only about situations when, in order to buy new sex for the price of marrying them, you consider breaking up with somebody you've been together with.

Just think how for us having rules against prostitution, this factual prostitution flourishes and thrives right before our eyes! Even celebrities brag about being in fact prostitutes, all across the media!

But you don't! Just respect your own integrity and don't!

And then, **I never complain about the weather**. There is no such a thing for me as bad weather. I am always too busy doing something cheerful. I always have so many exciting things going on. I am in love. How is it possible not to feel joy even when the weather is wet, dark, slushy! Apart of that, the small tower top lights look so beautiful in this type of weather. And the fire in the furnace is the most enjoyable just then.

Love As The Core Attitude

When I was only taking my first steps into the learning of how to live my life with integrity, I had to face and answer for myself the question whether I wanted to love those whom I love or just own them. And I made up my mind. I chose to love them and not own them.

Living with this attitude is an inseparable ingredient of my integrity, even the quintessence of it.

The Two Options

Whenever there comes an unexpected, entangled situation, I always ask myself before acting, whether the way I act would support my integrity or damage it. I always choose to act in a way that supports my integrity.

People who consciously choose integrity know how it feels. Integrity is their normal state. Those people value their freedom. You can't buy them. You can't buy their opinion for money because they stick to the values that are far beyond what can be bought for money. You can't bribe them even with very big money.

They know that those who lose the personal integrity, they lose, in fact, everything. They lose their life. Love and joy can't flow. They can't see the joy that exists in those small, simple things that are always around us. They need bigger and bigger things to impress them, and they have never enough. And that is a tragedy, indeed. They think they are living, but in fact they are not. They are just slaves of what they own.

Restoring your personal integrity is a home task, a mandatory step before you take on any therapy, any health improvement project. Nothing will give you a sustainable result if your integrity is damaged.

First restore your integrity, only then go and visit the doctor.

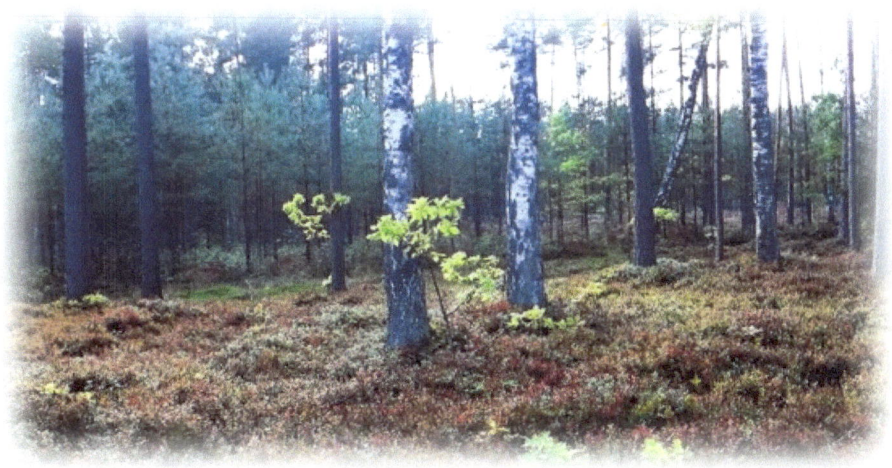

Questions For Self Check

1. Do you have full and unconditional acceptance of your own self?

It is not enough if you are happy with yourself by 99%. Only undoubted 100% qualifies.

Prof. Mirzakarim Norbekov in his book "The Experience Of A Fool Who Had An Epiphany About How To Get Rid Of His Glasses" gives the following mental picture.

If in a range from 0 to 100, your acceptance of yourself is 99, and dissatisfaction is 1, then your life looks like a food made from 99 parts of honey and 1 part of cyanide.

100% of self acceptance is not a target. It is, in fact, the absolute requirement for everybody who wants to live with integrity and enjoy the good fruit thereof. 100% of self acceptance is not a value that can wait until you reach it gradually. It needs to be TAKEN here and now. Living one more minute with incomplete self acceptance is already too much.

100% of self acceptance is a decision that needs to be taken immediately. This is the right moment to decide. And then you need to repeat it for yourself until it sinks well into your subconscious. You are wonderful, and all the components in you are wonderfully made.

You did not buy yourself. You did not make yourself. You were wonderfully made in your Mother's belly, you were kept growing, all your bones, sinews, organs - proportionally.

Are you humble enough to see that the yourself is actually a precious, invaluable, extremely complex GIFT to yourself? Consequently, that is none of your business to be satisfied with yourself or not. 100% is the only figure available for you to choose. "Excellent" is the only mark available for giving to yourself.

But if you create for yourself ranges with values less than 100% , if you create marks lower than "Excellent", then you are, in fact, meaning offense to the Origin that gave the yourself to you! Have you ever considered that? Are you humble enough to recognize that?

Full and unconditional self acceptance is determined by the independent reality in which we all exist. Full and unconditional self acceptance is, in fact, a sign of true humbleness. It is a sign of you being in conformity with the independent reality. Nothing more. And nothing less.

2. Are your thoughts, words and actions in alignment?

If they are not, then let this very minute be the very last in the whole life of yours when they were not. From this very moment, please take good care to keep your thoughts, words and actions in alignment.

If you sabotage yourself, if you are not one whole person with yourself, then there is no use of doing anything. There is no doctor in the whole world who would be able to help you.

3. Are you free from guilt, real or inspired?

Sense of guilt can turn our life into a hell. Sense of guilt blocks all joy, makes us feel wretched. Sense of guilt is used by ideologies and religions as the main tool of keeping people as their followers or paying customers.

Sense of guilt can be real or imaginary.

Real guilt has to be dealt with. It can be truly bad things that haunt you. But you have only one life and only two options. You may repent, which means that you admit the wrongdoings to your own self and decide that it was wrong to do them. However harsh the crime, when you admit it and regret it, it is all you can do and all you need to do. Then you only need to leave it in the past.

Yes, it was you who did it. You can't have it undone. But you must not allow it to destroy the whole life of yours. You have learned your lesson, let it be enough. You are now a different person. You are now more balanced, more open to love, and wiser, after all.

If you feel bad about the past wrongs you have committed, if you feel you would never again stoop to anything of that kind, then you are free. Now only don't torture yourself with memories. Direct your thoughts forward. Allow yourself to be free, to be a new person. Yes, there may be the real world consequences of

The other option is not to admit, not to repent and continue to carry your guilt for the rest of your life like an iron ball chained to your leg. You are free to choose so. Only then don't have any expectations. Joy of life, true pleasure, happiness, those things are simply not for you then. But you decide. I personally don't know how anyone would choose the second option. In the real life, however, I see people choosing it again, again and again.

But if your guilt is not real, just imaginary, just inspired, then drop it now. Don't carry it one more minute. Drop it! Now is the right time!

Too many people consider themselves guilty for even being born. Usually because some religion or cult has inspired that idea.

I met a Mother the other day, whose baby child was diagnosed with some inherited problem. "I feel guilty for not being able even to give birth to a healthy child," said she.

I hardly believed I was hearing that. How can such a thinking pattern be even possible? How can she be responsible and guilty for something like that, for something that is completely beyond her control? But again, again and again I see the same thinking pattern in people. They ruin their integrity with this kind of ideas, and they suffer.

I think this attitude should be stopped right here and right now! Just start living your life! Never feel responsible or even guilty for things that you can't control. You are responsible only for the things that you can control. You can be guilty only for the wrong decisions and actions of yours.

Number One Source Of Guilt

But the number one source of guilt, the absolute winner in making billions of people feel guilty and miserable is - sex. People feel guilty not only for wanting or doing, but also for just thinking of it. Can you believe such is possible in the modern world? But, however sadly, it is, and all too frequently.

I don't want to dwell on this subject more than it is absolutely necessary for the scope of this material. The one thing that, for the sake of our integrity, we need to understand very well is the fact that sex is a normal natural need, source of matchless joy and a wonderful gift from whoever created us, call it God if you like. Believe me or not, sex can be highly enjoyable and give you a lot of pleasure, happiness and the most pleasant memories for the rest of your life.

We label sex, undeservedly, with all the worst words we know. We should, instead, be happy and grateful. We should treat it as the most precious gift and learn to truly enjoy it rather than frown at it. It helps us to survive harsh times. It makes people kinder and happier.

People need hugs and caressing touches. People need orgasm now and then, too. Most people with very few exceptions need it regardless of their marital status. And to have it is their birthright.

Most people like it, want it, dream of it and long for it. And, however sad, when they take an action to get it, they feel guilty. They feel guilty, in fact, for being humans, do they not?

The sense of guilt for sex that too many people carry on themselves is an imaginary guilt, an inspired guilt. It does not need any repentance at all.

If you are serious about living with integrity, just drop that guilt right here and now. Never hold yourself or any other person guilty for sex as long as it is used for its natural purpose of giving and getting pleasure and relief, and does not insult, harm or cause damage to anyone.

4. Is love your unquestionable attitude towards absolutely all the people of the world, including your own self?

Love in this context is an attitude that wishes all and everybody well, and readiness to contribute if their well-being gets dependent on you.

If you love all the people except just one, then you can visualize yourself chained by just one strong chain in a place where there tide waters are soon expected. You are on chain, and a question how to live a healthier, more fulfilling life is pointless.

You need first to break free from all your chains. Only then you can think of improvement for your health or overall wellness.

But what if you have a few people whom you hate, whom you can't forgive, for whom you nourish thoughts of retaliation?

No worries whatsoever! That is just an attitude, after all. Just take a brave decision and change it right here and now, and go happy and free.

There is nothing more to that, indeed.

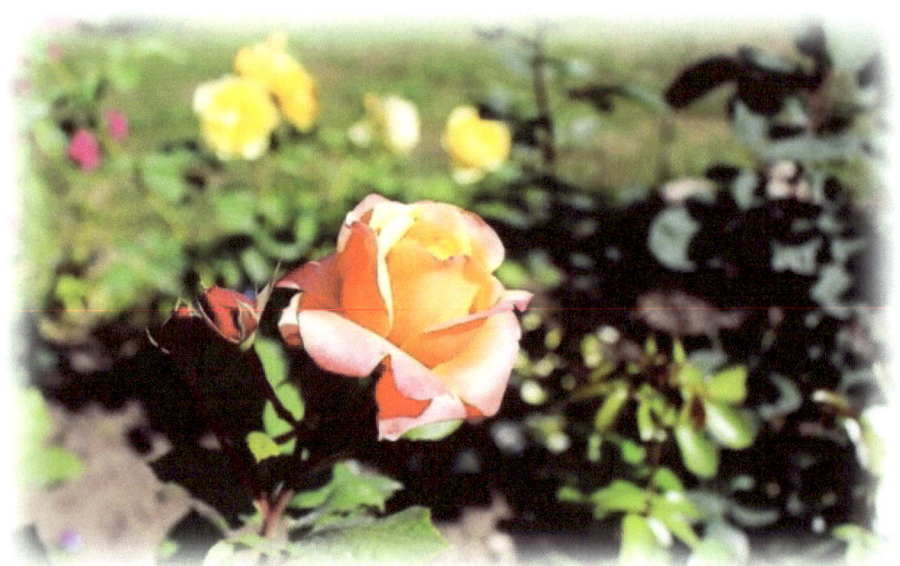

Three Steps To Integrity

The following is my attempt to present the whole story in a few actionable steps. I did those steps many years ago, and I feel that that is the best favor I have ever done to myself.

1. Define Love as the unquestionable attitude towards my own self, other people and the reality on the whole. Love in this context means wishing everyone happiness, being ready to help generously and free of charge in situations when they might need such help.

This is only a decision and should not take more than two seconds to take. Don't waste your valuable time, indeed. Just decide for yourself, and that is all there is to it.

2. Forgive everything, including even all the future wrongs. Forgiving in this context means allowing yourself to be free from obligation to hate the wrong doer, think and rethink the wrongs, retaliate.

Forgiving does not mean forgetting, removing the responsibility from the guilty person, hugging or kissing the wrong doer. It just means freeing yourself from the obligation to victimize yourself, to continue re-suffering of the wrong by thinking of it again and again.

Forgiving is just a decision, too. Two seconds from your life should be more than enough to take it and start living it.

3. Align your behavior, your thoughts, words and deeds with those decisions. From now on, live your life consistently in accordance with those decisions.

This is by far the most difficult step. Unlike the earlier, this is not a decision but a process. It may take some time and effort before you feel that your subconscious attitudes have changed.

If you, for example, have been calling yourself an idiot for a certain period of time, then now you must get out of that habit. You have decided to love yourself. But it is not always easy to get rid from all the junk practices that you have used against yourself through years. An idea like "I need to be slim to be loved" is a junk. It will have to be replaced with something healthy, like "I am wonderful, loving and lovable just as I am and because I am".

If you have been starving yourself on joy, pleasure, movement, then you will have to stop that immediately. You must start seeing joy in small things, you must allow yourself pleasure and be grateful for it, you must move a lot and cheerfully. Yes, it is of critical importance that you move cheerfully. Allow being in movement to be your very source of your cheerful mood. And allow your cheerful mood find its fulfillment in moving.

And, above all, there is gratefulness.

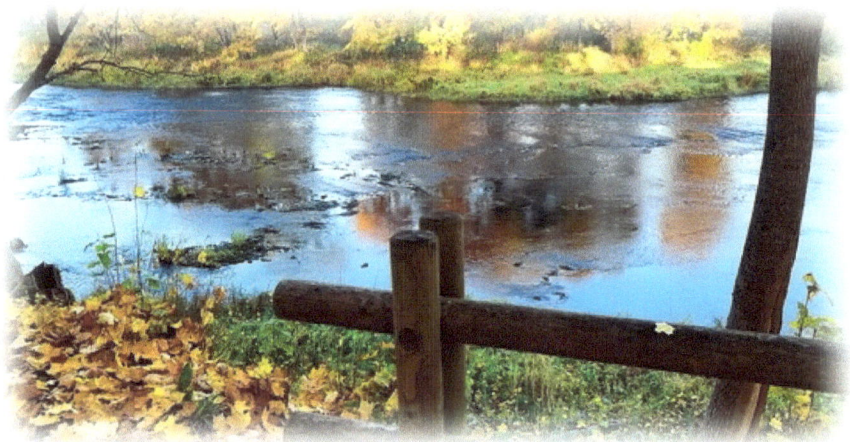

How I Benefit From Living With Integrity

All the things that I describe here I also live by on daily basis. Having tasted once this simple way of living and being well, I have made up my mind. I want no other way.

Whenever I would feel tempted to sell my integrity for money, like for giving a corrupt opinion, I don't fall for that. And not because I would be a good boy or a very ethical citizen. I have simply got to taste and see for myself how enjoyable can be life if you live it being a whole person, if you live with integrity.

Whenever I would receive an offer to sell my integrity in one way or the other, it is easy for me to reject it. I have an easy trick to keep me always on the safe side.

I just see very clearly that my life consists of moments. And it is beyond my control how many of them I will be given in my life. I can't be even sure about my tomorrow or even about my next few seconds. So, whatever amount you offer me, let it be even billions, I always remember to multiply with the number of moments within my control, and that is Zero.

That is an easy calculation, is it not? No matter how much you offer, it will always be only me selling myself. But what I actually get, will always be Zero. Is this too weak an argument for staying uncorrupted, staying with integrity?

The reason for living with integrity should never be based on the expectancies of others. It is yourself who benefits from it the most. Just consider some of these:

» Constant being in love with life carries me like on wings.

» Simple things give me joy.

» I have courage to speak what I feel.

» My ups are high up, my downs are never too deep.

» I have tight, sound sleep at night. I never have problems with getting sleep. No nightmares ever bother me.

» I have great health even though I did nothing to have it, other than just reclaiming my integrity. When I did, I felt myself healing. Practically all my health issues are gone since then. I have had no virus for around nine years, and that coincides with the time when I took the decision to live on as a man of integrity. Heavy headaches that I used to have like once or twice a week are all gone long since. I don't even remember how it feels when you have headache.

» I am much more efficient in whatever I do, and all my efforts are much more rewarding.

Well, there are some downsides, too. I feel that I am now a difficult person for a larger number of people than before. Some people get resentful. I think mostly because they don't believe that the same degree of wellness is readily available for them, too. I believe, however, that most of them do see what is possible even for them. Only they are too irresolute to cut all the strings that tie them up and make them into factual slaves.

Integrity requires determination and courage, that is true. But when you think of the reward, and that is nothing less than the life well lived, then it suddenly gets very easy to decide.

Don'ts

» **Never use living with integrity as a means for achieving something else** like health, slim body, financial success, improved relations, etc. Living with integrity is a supreme value in itself. Personal integrity is always the reason for itself. To live with integrity is the only way of living the life well. Whenever you try to use your integrity as a pill or slimming program – guess what – you lose it right there.

Integrity is integrity only when it exists for no reason other than integrity itself. The moment you start manipulating it, you lose it. Period.

On the other hand, living with integrity will most likely clean most of your health issues, even the long term ones, even without your focusing. It did for me, in any case.

» **Never have integrity related expectations**.

A friend of mine asked me once: "What if you were diagnosed with cancer some day, and so your method proved wrong?"

First of all, this is not a method.

This is just a very firm and secure as can be foundation. On this foundation, you can test and try any method, any therapy, any plan. And – guess what – they are likely to work. Whatever you undertake is much more likely to work and bear fruit on this solid foundation than on the quick sand of something else.

So for example, if your environment is healthy, then also your walk will be more enjoyable and beneficial for your health. If the operating system on your device is good, then your applications will run smoothly.

More to that, it may turn out that you need no therapies or methods whatsoever. In my case, I felt myself healing right from the moment when I took the decision to live the rest of my life with integrity. My way up began right from the point of taking that decision.

But, as is understood, nothing can be safe and predictable by 100%. Am I still vulnerable? Yes, I am. I am as exposed to all kinds of troubles as anyone else. Only when you live with integrity, you are much better prepared.

When you live with integrity, you may still be in pain, you may still fall sick occasionally. But your being one and united within yourself will make you strong. You will be able to feel joy and happiness in spite of whatever the troubles. You will suffer much less. The recovery will be much faster. Even the most hopeless things may start yielding the treatment and may even go over all by themselves.

Well, there is a great method that has always worked for me. Yes, it needs your personal integrity as the basis. Give yourself regular "injections" of joy! Remember your happiest moments, visualize those that you would eagerly want to experience!

Don't care the least that those thoughts may be wild, untamed, frowned at by 98% of the population.

Only these thoughts must exclude all the evil, be completely free from hate, revenge, hurting others. Such things can't give joy. But if you do feel joy by visualizing of something like that, then, I'm afraid, you need a serious expert help.

But think happy, cheerful, kind thoughts. Allow joy to flow in abundance. Celebrate the amazing reality in which you live.

Works for me incredibly well, and will most certainly work for you, too.

» **Never use positive thinking**. It is dangerous. It is deceptive and guilt inspiring. I never use positive thinking, and even if it may sound at times that I do, that is not true. I use **real thinking**. Real thinking has a tremendous power in it because it is true, it is reality based and it is independent from man's will.

Real thinking gives me a lot of positive emotions that strengthen me, heal me, entertain me.

Positive thinking is something for people who do not have courage or determination to live their integrity. Let them continue finding their "silver lining" in otherwise depressing things.

But people with integrity thrive even on negative emotions. They feel stable and prepared having done their negative visualization of the challenges that they need to face.

I personally use negative visualization a lot. It boosts dramatically my ability to appreciate what I have now. It fosters gratefulness in me.

But gratefulness is the key of – everything.

Where I Get Courage From

» Above all is gratefulness. I feel grateful for being alive. But I also think a lot about death. I always remind myself about my being mortal. I think of the current moment like of something valuable that needs to be lived. I foster in me awareness that I have no control over my moments. And that is how I feel even more grateful for what I have here and now. This gratefulness gives me peace of mind and courage.

» I remind myself often that this very moment can be my last one on this planet. I ask myself a question whether I would worry about the same things if I knew that this current day were my last one. And it can very well be, too. I ask myself what I would do then. It gives me courage to seize the present moment, to celebrate it and to act bravely and resolutely.

» I nourish the awareness in me that I am wonderfully made. I did not make myself or buy myself. There is some great Master who has made me into what I am. So I only assume the part of responsibility for how I keep myself. But the part of the responsibility for how I am made, I shift to that invisible, unknown Master, the same One, who has made even you. Not carrying responsibility for the things that I can't be responsible for, gives me courage.

» Being in love is a very powerful source of courage. I have to confess, I used to feel guilty for being in love. You can understand that, can't you? There are two many factors all around that teach us to feel guilty – schools, religions, rules, media, even our own friends and family at times.

Now I see being in love as a value. I consciously train myself to be in love as often as possible, and I target to make this state constant.

There is no other thing in the whole world that can come even close to being in love. The joy that it gives me is overwhelming.

It is easy to be brave, it is easy to be strong, it is easy to face challenges when you are in love!

My target is to be in love all of the time, and I feel I am doing better and better. And you?

Egil Nelius

The One Last Word

Gratefulness.

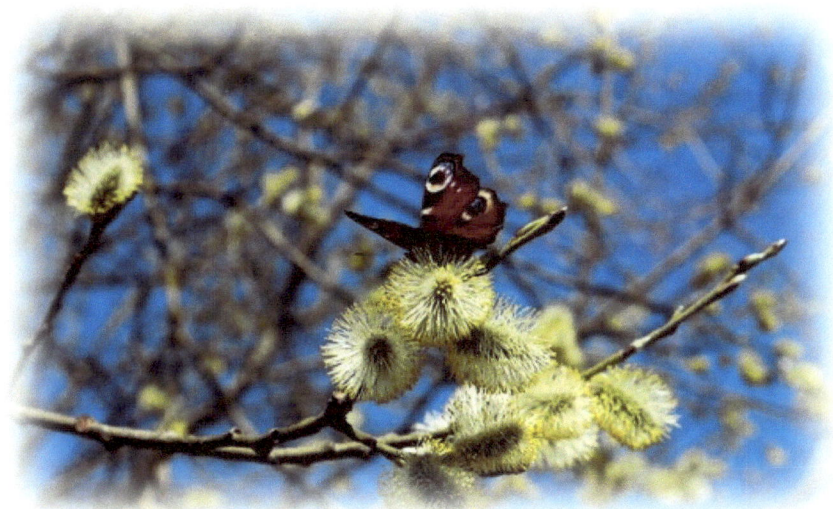

Resources

The Strange Joy – author's website

Integrity - Wikipedia

Psychology Today. 7 Signs Of People With Integrity

Global Leadership: True Meaning Of Integrity

Kahlil Gibran. "The Prophet"

Mirzakarim Norbekov. "The experience of a fool: who had an epiphany about how to get rid of his glasses"

Christopher McDougall. "Born To Run"

ACE: How To Find The JOY In Exercise

Lessons From The Samurai: The Secret To Always Being At Your Best

4 Lifehacks From Ancient Philosophers That Will Make You Happier

Integrity Quotes

Egil Nelius

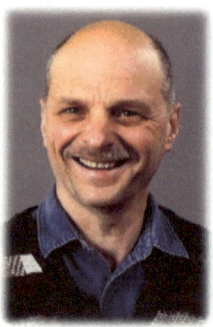

About The Author

Egil Nelius, born in 1963, is a Latvian teacher, webmaster, DIY man, hobby artist, outdoor goer, husband, father of 5, enthusiast of values based living.

In the recent years, Egil has learned a lot about the healing power and other benefits that can be found in reality connected living. By mindful observation of the independent reality and drawing well grounded conclusions thereof, he has given himself a second chance to feel joy, love and true happiness.

Apart of that, he has had his once critically poor health completely restored to a level of never before experienced stable healthiness.

Egil loves to speak and write about the different aspects of his experience. He does that in a patient, friendly manner, because he can't think of a better reward than seeing other people get happier.

Once a lady of 84 said: "Egil, nobody has ever spoken to me like this! What a life I would have lived if they had done!"

His answer was: "Then now you have only two options to choose from: you can either continue as you did so far, or you can start, from this very moment onwards, celebrating your moments as they are still being given to you!"

Egil believes also that by exploring the amazing reality around us, we can get to know a lot about its Creator.

Visit Egil's website at thestrangejoy.com .

Egil Nelius

Design by Egil Nelius

Photographs: Egil and Dag Nelius